CREATE ANEWU HEALTH MINISTRY

Presents
How To Lose Weight Fast

Learning to eat your way to ANEWU!

Then God said,
"I give you every seed-bearing plant
On the face of the whole earth
And every tree that has fruit with seed in it.
They will be yours for food."

Genesis 1:29

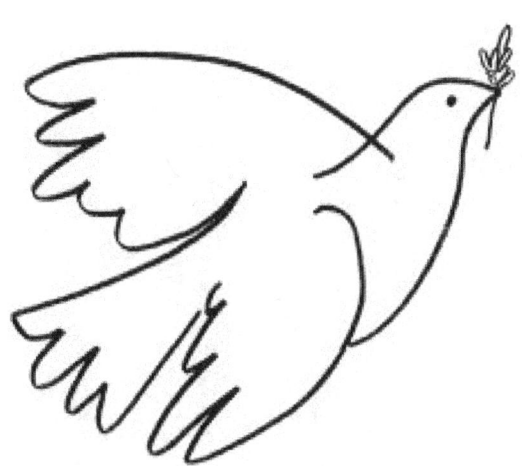

Dr. Kathleen B. Oden
Certified Health Minister

Table of Contents

CREATE ANEWU HEALTH MINISTRY

Beloved,
I wish above all things
that thou mayest prosper
and be in health,
even as thy soul prospereth.
3 JOHN 1:2

PREFACE

This is a Bible based, weight loss plan. Even Jesus said in John 5:30,

"I can of mine own self do nothing: as I hear,
I judge: and my judgment is just;
because I seek not mine own will,
but the will of the Father which hath sent me."

The information in this book is based on Biblical principles in the Holy Bible. And like Jesus, we cannot do it, on our own. Therefore, before starting this journey, please pray and ask the Holy Spirit for guidance, because you will need HIM every step of the way.

But seek ye first the kingdom of God,
and his righteousness;
and all these things shall be added unto you.
Matthew 6:33

It is not easy to change your entire way of eating. This is not a diet, but a life changing decision and experience. This journey started out fun and exciting, then, it became hard and boring. But now, I no longer look at food the same way, because now this is a mission for me to rebuild the temple of God.

I feel like Solomon and Nehemiah. Their mission was to build and rebuild. Your mission is to build and rebuild. Forget about yourself and think about how much you love God and how much you want HIM to live in a palace and not a pit. You can do this! Now Repeat...

I can do all things through Christ which strengtheneth me.
Philippians 4:13

INTRODUCTION

If you are struggling with being overweight, then this book is for you. The information in this book will give you the knowledge you need to learn the right way to not only, lose weight, but to also get healthy.

The 21 Day Weight Loss Challenge, will jump-start your weight loss and put you on the fast track to learning how to eat healthy to lose weight and be healthy. Losing weight is not going to help you if you are not also, healthy. No one wants to be skinny if that also means being sickly.

Please feel free to use the website in conjunction with this book as well as email. I am always glad to consult with you. If you would like access to my recipes, please email me for that information.

Since I am a minister, I am also here to pray for you and with you. Please contact me if you need prayer. I pray that God be with you on this journey as He is with me.

O come, let us worship and bow down:
let us kneel before the LORD our maker.
Psalm 95:6

DEDICATION & ACKNOWLEDGMENTS

I dedicate this book and give all glory and honor to the

True and Living God,
And to my
Lord and Savior, Jesus Christ,
And the
Holy Spirit,

for giving me the mindset and strength, to write this book:

21 Day Weight Loss Challenge
& How To Lose Weight Fast

I thank God and acknowledgment and dedicate this book to, My Apostle

Dr. Dorothy J. Page

For her dedication to my spiritual growth.
I love you and thank God for the spiritual guidance & teaching
that you have imparted to my life.
Your life has inspired me to continue to live for God
and do the work which He has called me to do.

I thank God and acknowledge My Sister In Christ,

Sis. Pamela Lavonne Barton

For her friendship, prayers, tears, love and support.
May God continue to bless you,
for helping me to edit this book for publishing.

REBUILDING THE TEMPLE
Repair the walls and guard the gates!

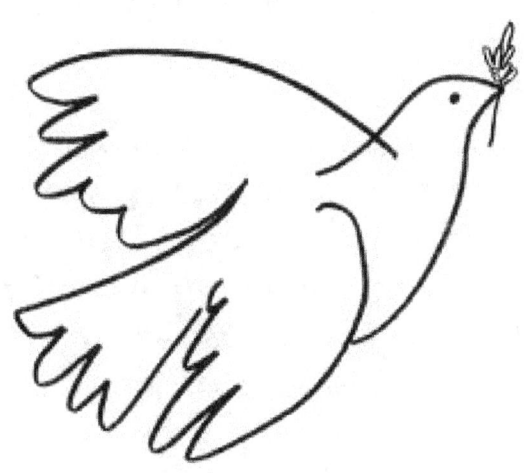

Humble yourselves therefore
under the mighty hand of God,
that he may exalt you in due time:
Casting all your care upon him;
for he careth for you.
1 Peter 5:6-7

REBUILDING THE TEMPLE
Repair the walls and guard the gates!

In order to do this, in order to repair the walls, we must first, guard the gates. And the main gate, is our mouth. And, we cannot repair the walls, (of our body/temple), if we do not have the right tools we need, to make the repairs. Therefore, we must return to God's original foundation plan for all mankind. His plan works for EVERYONE...

29 And God said, Behold,
I have given you every herb yielding seed,
which is upon the face of all the earth, and every tree,
in which is the fruit of a tree yielding seed;
to you it shall be for food:
GENESIS 1:29

And why call ye me, Lord, Lord,
and do not the things which I say?
47 Whosoever cometh to me, and heareth my sayings,
and doeth them, I will shew you to whom he is like:
48 He is like a man which built an house, and digged deep, and laid the
foundation on a rock: and when the flood arose, the stream beat
vehemently upon that house, and could not shake it: for it was founded
upon a rock.   LUKE 6:46-48

Before the flood, plants were man's only diet. But all living things died during the flood.

"And every living substance was destroyed which was upon the face of the ground..."

GENESIS 7:23

Therefore, there was not enough plants for man to eat and survive. This is why God tells Noah to add meat to his diet, and, that man and animals, will no longer live in harmony...

And God blessed Noah and his sons, and said unto them, Be fruitful, and multiply, and replenish the earth. And the fear of you and the dread of you shall be upon every beast of the earth, and upon every bird of the heavens; With all wherewith the ground teemeth, and all the fishes of the sea, into your hand are they delivered. Every moving thing that liveth shall be food for you; As the green herb have I given you all.
GENESIS 9:1-3

However, we can see (by the last line in verse 3), that God did not abolish His original foundation plan for man. When God brought the children of Israel out of Egypt, He tried to wean them off the meat, that they were used to eating in Egypt. But the children of Israel, were not happy with the plant based MANNA diet, that God gave them.

Lets face it, most people love meat. And once man started eating animal flesh, he did not want to stop. Man become addicted to animal flesh. In fact, the children of Israel murmured and complained, because they would rather be dead, then to stop eating animal flesh...

And the whole congregation of the children of Israel murmured against Moses and Aaron in the wilderness: 3 And the children of Israel said unto them, Would to God we had died by the hand of the LORD in the land of Egypt, when we sat by the flesh pots, and did eat bread to the full; for ye have brought us forth into this wilderness, to kill this whole assembly with hunger. EXODUS 16:3

_____

_____

_____

Today, some people feel the same way. They would rather be dead, then to eat healthy, and live a healthy life. Does this mean, people must totally give up eating meat? No! Does this mean that people have to eat boring or terrible tasting food, in order to eat healthy? No, again! The children of Israel, did not stop complaining. They continued to murmur and complain, until God gave them meat. But he also gave them death...

PSALM 78:22-32

Because they believed not in God, and trusted not in his salvation: 23 Though he had commanded the clouds from above, and opened the doors of heaven, 24 And had rained down manna upon them to eat, and had given them of the corn of heaven. 25 Man did eat angels' food: he sent them meat to the full. 26 He caused an east wind to blow in the heaven: and by his power he brought in the south wind.

27 He rained flesh also upon them as dust, and feathered fowls like as the sand of the sea: 28 And he let it fall in the midst of their camp, round about their habitations. 29 So they did eat, and were filled: for he gave them their own desire; 30 They were not estranged from their lust. But while their meat was yet in their mouths, 31 The wrath of God came upon them, and slew the fattest of them, and smote down the chosen men of Israel. 32 For all this they sinned still, and believed not for his wondrous works.

_____

_____

_____

_____

_____

_____

Some people are convinced that "man" cannot survive without eating meat. But we can see, that is not true. Because most of the people that eat meat, are not healthy. They are sickly and over weight. However, very few vegans or vegetarians are sickly and/or over weight.

The real truth is, man cannot survive, by continuing to eat a lot of meat. In America, people are eating so much meat, the animals are drinking more water then humans. How is this possible? It is possible, because animals also have to eat. And whether they eat corn or wheat or whatever, it also, has to be watered, in order to grow.

So the majority of the water in the U.S. is used for animals and their food. You would think, humans would be more important than animals. But due to the amount of meat consumed in America, more than half of the water in this country, goes to raise more and more animals, for meat consumption.

It only takes 49 gallons of water to grow a pound of apples and 24 gallons, for a pound of potatoes. But it takes approximately 5000 gallons of water per, 1 pound of beef. 80% of corn grown in the U.S. is eaten by animals and 90% of the soy and oats. That means that high amounts of herbicides and fungicides are used at farms, including nitrate fertilizers, pesticides and antibiotics. Those drugs are then passed down to the meat and dairy products that people consume. And some of these chemicals can now also be found in our lakes, streams and water ways, killing the fish and plant life.

And that ye may put difference between holy and unholy,
and between unclean and clean
LEV 10:10

_____

_____

_____

_____

Most of the meat sold today is contaminated with chemicals. However, there are organic and kosher meats that are not contaminated. The body, can protect itself, if it receives more nutrients and less chemicals. Our bodies are only disease proof, when we don't abuse them.

Most people consume approximately 12 pounds of chemicals a year. We have to breath air, but we do not have to continue to consume certain foods, or use products that are loaded with chemicals. We can eat less: meat, fat, eggs and dairy and eat more whole grains, nuts, fruits and vegetables, then we can wean ourselves, little by little, until we lower the amount of chemicals in our body and raise the amount of nutrients. This will cause our body to reverse or stop, the destruct mode and causing the body to go into a healing mode. And over time, you will start to feel better, get stronger and live longer. **This is what it will take to Create Anewu!**

For I will restore health unto thee,
and I will heal thee of thy wounds...
JEREMIAH 30:17

And Jesus saith unto him,
I will come and heal him.
MATTHEW 8:7

_____

_____

_____

_____

_____

My **CREATE ANEWU** program, will give you the support that you need, in order to turn your health around. There are very few people or even Christians, that can say, "I have good or excellent health." No one, has to be sick, no one has to be tired and no one has to be over weight.

But, we do have to be committed to God and committed to rebuilding our temple. God wants us to be healthy. Taking care of the temple of God is very important. If someone gave us a brand new building to have our Church service, we would go all out, to take care of it and we would buy the best of everything to put into it. But God does not live in a building, He lives in us. We, are His real home, His real temple. We must commit to buying the best food to not only rebuild it, but also to maintain it.

Beloved, I wish above all things that thou mayest prosper
and be in health, even as thy soul prospereth.
3 JOHN 1:2

What?
know ye not that your body is the temple of the Holy Ghost which
is in you, which ye have of God,
and ye are not your own?
For ye are bought with a price:
therefore glorify God in your body,
and in your spirit, which are God's.
1 CORINTHIANS 6:19

It's Time To Create Anewu!

createanewuhealthministry.com

HOW TO USE THIS BOOK

To get the best results from this book, please follow these instructions. Before starting on the 21 DAY CHALLENGE, please read the following in this order, after you have read, REBUILDING THE TEMPLE:

"KNOWLEDGE IS POWER"

Therefore, you need to gain the knowledge you need, in order to successfully lose, the amount of weight you want or need, to lose. How To Lose Weight Fast, will teach you not only the fastest way to lose weight, but also, the safest.

You also need to learn What & How Much To Eat, so that you will get all the vitamins, minerals and nutrients that you need. The 3 Food Groups will teach you about the different types of food as well as, what is "NOT FOOD".

Learning how to get rid of the Top 5 Killers, is your biggest hurdle and will cause dramatic weight loss, if you can do it. Creating Anewu and How Enzymes Work, will teach you how the cells in your body work with the enzymes in your body, to help rebuild your body. Read and learn.

HOW TO LOSE WEIGHT FAST

The fastest way to lose weight fast is to eat every 2-3 hours. The first time I heard that, I thought they were crazy. But since I love to eat, that was no problem for me. And, after I tried it, I realized ok, this is working. I was losing about 2-3 pounds a week or 10-12 pounds a month. And in 3 months, I had lost 40 pounds.

I ate from 8am to 8pm, however, I did eat breakfast and lunch, because I was still working at the time, not retired. But by the time I went home at 4pm, I was so full, I did not want to see any food. But I continued to eat, because it is very important to eat every 2 hours.

8AM	-	bottle of water
10AM	-	bottle of water
12PM	-	salad
2PM	-	bottle of water
4PM	-	soup
6PM	-	fruit smoothie
8PM	-	snack

I learned that our body automatically looks for food every 2-3 hours. We have to "trick" the body so that it will not go into "I'm hungry mode" by sending a signal to your brain that tells you to go eat.

Eating every 2-3 hours will put a stop to the "I'm hungry mode" and it will cause your body to go into the "fat burning mode." When we eat every 2-3 hours, our body says, "ok cells, unlock the fat and let it go and hurry up and get rid of all this food that keeps coming in here."

Our body starts working overtime and triple time to get rid of fat as fast as it can. But the trick is, What & How Much To Eat.

WHAT & HOW MUCH TO EAT

I can only recommend or make suggestions on what and/or how much you are to eat. You will have to make your own plan, using the plans below, as an example.

You should try to eat all big meals before 3pm. After 3pm eat soup, smoothies and snacks. Try not to drink anything after 3pm. Try to keep your total calorie intake to 1200 calories, a day and take vitamins.

8AM	-	bottle of water
10AM	-	bottle of water
12PM	-	large salad
2PM	-	bottle of water
4PM	-	1/2 cup soup with 3 crackers
6PM	-	green smoothie
8PM	-	snack (carrot sticks, celery sticks...etc)

8AM	-	breakfast & bottle of water
10AM	-	snack
12PM	-	lunch & bottle of water
2PM	-	bottle of water
4PM	-	snack (carrot sticks, celery sticks...etc)
6PM	-	fruit smoothie
8PM	-	1/2 cup soup with 3 crackers

THE 3 FOOD GROUPS

Living Foods
Living foods are raw uncooked foods. They are the most powerful, they have the most vitamins and nutrients. Eat raw foods everyday.

Dead Foods
All Cooked foods. Cooked food has very little or no vitamins or nutrients alive in it. Steamed food is better. Eat cooked foods 2-3 days a week.

Toxic Foods
Anything that has chemicals added to it to preserve it, color it, or make it look or taste good...etc. This is not food, but pure poison. Eat this no more than 2-3 days a month. Try to eliminate completely.

This is my favorite salad:

lettuce - 3 leaves

spinach - 3 leaves

collard greens -3 leaves

kale - 3 leaves

tomato - 1

green onion - 2

jalapeno - 1

grapes - 10

After I eat this salad, I feel strong and energized, for the rest of the day. I don't feel weighted down or thirsty. No salt or sugar cravings. No urges to make wrong food choices. It balances out my day.

This salad also keeps me regulated throughout the week. It is quick and easy to make and very portable. The green onion makes it smell yummy and inviting. The jalapeno gives it a spicy kick and the grapes make it sweet and juicy. YUM!

NOTES

THE TOP 5 KILLERS

1- Meat and meat by products: Eggs, milk & cheese
2 - sugar
3 - white flour
4 - salt
5 - caffeine

Americans are slowly poisoning themselves, and some of them have absolutely, no idea, that these items contain lethal, deadly, poison chemicals and toxins.

High amounts of herbicides and fungicides are used at farms, including nitrate fertilizers, pesticides and antibiotics. Those drugs are then passed down to the meat and dairy products that people consume. And some of these chemicals can now also be found in our lakes, streams and water ways, killing the fish and plant life.

Sugar pulls large amounts of calcium from the bones in the body, which causes the bones and teeth to decay. Eating large amounts of sugar can causes asthma, arthritis and nervous disorders to name a few.

When lab rats are fed white flour, they die in a week to 10 days. White flour is bleached, preserved and aged with Chlorine Dioxide. This helps white bread to continue to look good, (for at least 2 weeks)when it is actually already rotten.

Eating large amounts of salt can lead to hardening of the arteries, kidney disease, congestive heart failure and more. Most people consume about 4000 mg. of salt per day, but the body can only handle about 2400 mg. per day.

Caffeine reduces the amount of oxygen that flows to the brain and other parts of the body by about 30%. This causes the digestive system and the immune system to become impaired.

NOTES

_____

_____

_____

_____

_____

_____

_____

_____

_____

_____

_____

_____

_____

_____

_____

_____

Creating Anewu!

People may think it is impossible to create a new you, but it can be done. God created our bodies to automatically repair itself, (IF) we eat healthy foods. We know this is true because whenever we get a cut on our hand, it heals.

Our bodies work the same way, but on a higher level. However, if we do not eat healthy foods then our body does not have enough vitamins and nutrients to keep it in healing mode. Therefore, the body cannot protect itself from arthritis, high blood pressure, diabetes and other ailments, that start forming in the body.

Our body is made of millions and millions of cells. And the condition of the cells determines the condition of our body. If the cells are weak or damaged, then we are weak and sickly. However, we can create new stronger cells by eating foods that are packed with live enzymes.

The most powerful foods are the green leafy vegetables, like collard green, mustered greens, turnip greens, spinach and kale.

> *Every moving thing that liveth shall be meat for you;*
> *even as the green herb have I given you all things.*
> *Genesis 9:3*

The quickest way to create new cells is to drink these greens. Put them in a blender, with water and an apple or two. This green smoothie will go directly to your cells and start creating new stronger cells immediately.

The second best way is to chop up the greens and make a salad. Add your favorite veggies like tomatoes, cucumbers, or whatever you like on your salad.

This is the quickest way to regain your strength and energy, and also repair your immune system. However, this must be done in conjunction with eliminating **THE TOP 5 KILLERS** (page 13), from your diet.

Try to eat a small salad with every cooked meal, so that you will have living enzymes to help digest the cooked food. Most cooked food has very little enzymes or no enzymes at all.

As you eat less and less foods that contain nitrate fertilizers, pesticides, antibiotics, and other lethal toxic chemicals and poisons, and eat more and more fresh raw green leafy foods, your body will respond.

It all depends on how bad your health is and how much of the powerful green leafy vegetables you add to your diet. Your main goal is to lower the chemicals in your body (eat these less) and raise the vitamins and minerals in your body by eating these more.

NOTES

_____

_____

_____

_____

_____

_____

_____

_____

_____

_____

_____

How Enzymes Work

There are 3 types of Enzymes...

1. **Metabolic Enzymes**   -   give energy to the bodily functions.

2. **Digestive Enzymes** - are produced in the pancreas and are responsible for digesting food.

There are 3 main digestive enzymes:

A - AMYLASE ENZYMES: digest carbohydrates

Amylase enzymes are produced in the mouth and start to digest food right away. If a person eats food that does not have any amylase enzymes, the body will send or borrow some amylase enzymes to help digest the food before it passes to the stomach.

B - PROTEASE ENZYMES: digest protein

Pro-tease enzymes take over when the food reaches the stomach. However, if the food does not have any pro tease enzymes, the body will send or borrow some pro tease enzymes to help digest the food before it passes to the small intestine.

C - LIPEASE ENZYMES: digest fat

If a person does not have enough lip-ease enzymes, when the body reaches the small intestines, the body will send or borrow some lip ease enzymes to help digest the fat.

3. **Food Enzymes** - are only present in raw foods. Cooked food has no enzymes. Therefore, cooked food just sits in the upper stomach until the body sends enzymes to digest it. The body will borrow metabolic enzymes (from wherever it can find them within the body), in order to digest cooked foods, thus preventing the body from completing normal bodily functions which can eventually lead to malfunction of the body.

NOTES

_____

_____

_____

_____

_____

_____

_____

_____

_____

_____

_____

_____

_____

_____

_____

_____

21 Day Weight Loss Challenge

Not unto us, O LORD, not unto us, but unto thy name give glory, for thy mercy, and for thy truth's sake. Psalm 115:1

21 Day Weight Loss Challenge

My goal is to lose _____ pounds

My current weight: _____ Date: _____

I completed the 21 Day Weight Loss Challenge and now I weigh:

_____

Other comments:

_____

_____

_____

_____

_____

_____

_____

_____

_____

WEEK 1

It you spend the first week of your 21 Day Weight Loss Challenge, renewing your love and commitment to God, it will give you a good foundation for the rest of your new healthy eating lifestyle.

Read 1 Chronicles Chapter 22, and prepare your heart and soul to seek the Lord. He loves you and wants to be with you. And He wants to help you and strengthen you to build "ANEWU." But, you have to ask for HIS help.

Give me understanding, and I shall keep thy law;
yea, I shall observe it with my whole heart.
Psalm 119:34

NOTES

_____

_____

_____

_____

_____

_____

_____

DAY 1

21 Day Weight Loss Challenge
SAMPLE Status Report

8AM   -   bottle of water

10AM   -   bottle of water

12PM   -   salad

2PM   -   bottle of water

4PM   -   soup

6PM   -   fruit smoothie

8PM   -   snack

_____

_____

_____

_____

_____

_____

DAY 1

21 Day Weight Loss Challenge   -   Status Report

_____

_____

_____

_____

_____

_____

_____

_____

_____

_____

_____

_____

_____

_____

_____

DAY 2

21 Day Weight Loss Challenge
SAMPLE Status Report

8AM   -   bottle of water

10AM   -   bottle of water

12PM   -   salad

2PM   -   bottle of water

4PM   -   soup

6PM   -   green smoothie

8PM   -   snack

_____

_____

_____

_____

_____

_____

_____

DAY 2

21 Day Weight Loss Challenge   -   Status Report

_____

_____

_____

_____

_____

_____

_____

_____

_____

_____

_____

_____

_____

_____

_____

_____

_____

DAY 3

21 Day Weight Loss Challenge
SAMPLE Status Report

8AM   -   bottle of water

10AM   -   bottle of water

12PM   -   salad

2PM   -   bottle of water

4PM   -   soup

6PM   -   fruit smoothie

8PM   -   snack

_____

_____

_____

_____

_____

_____

_____

DAY 3

21 Day Weight Loss Challenge   -   Status Report

_____

_____

_____

_____

_____

_____

_____

_____

_____

_____

_____

_____

_____

_____

_____

_____

_____

DAY 4

21 Day Weight Loss Challenge
SAMPLE Status Report

8AM   -   bottle of water

10AM   -   bottle of water

12PM   -   salad

2PM   -   bottle of water

4PM   -   soup

6PM   -   lemonade

8PM   -   snack

_____

_____

_____

_____

_____

_____

_____

DAY 4

21 Day Weight Loss Challenge - Status Report

_____

_____

_____

_____

_____

_____

_____

_____

_____

_____

_____

_____

_____

_____

_____

DAY 5

21 Day Weight Loss Challenge
SAMPLE Status Report

8AM   -   bottle of water

10AM   -   bottle of water

12PM   -   salad

2PM   -   bottle of water

4PM   -   soup

6PM   -   lemonade

8PM   -   snack

_____

_____

_____

_____

_____

_____

DAY 5

21 Day Weight Loss Challenge   -   Status Report

_____

_____

_____

_____

_____

_____

_____

_____

_____

_____

_____

_____

_____

_____

_____

DAY 6

21 Day Weight Loss Challenge
SAMPLE Status Report

8AM   -   bottle of water

10AM   -   bottle of water

12PM   -   small meal

2PM   -   bottle of water

4PM   -   salad

6PM   -   green smoothie

8PM   -   snack

_____

_____

_____

_____

_____

_____

_____

DAY 6

21 Day Weight Loss Challenge   -   Status Report

_____

_____

_____

_____

_____

_____

_____

_____

_____

_____

_____

_____

_____

_____

_____

_____

_____

DAY 7

21 Day Weight Loss Challenge
SAMPLE Status Report

8AM   -   bottle of water

10AM   -   bottle of water

12PM   -   small meal

2PM   -   bottle of water

4PM   -   salad

6PM   -   green smoothie

8PM   -   snack

_____

_____

_____

_____

_____

_____

_____

DAY 7

21 Day Weight Loss Challenge   -   Status Report

_____

_____

_____

_____

_____

_____

_____

_____

_____

_____

_____

_____

_____

_____

_____

WEEK 2

Spend week 2, praying for others on the 21 Day Challenge, as well as, your family, friends and other people. As you begin to focus on others and not on the 21 Day Challenge, the time will go by much faster.

Build a prayer list that you can continue to use on a daily basis. Read 1 Kings Chapter 8

But verily God hath heard me;
he hath attended to the voice of my prayer.
Blessed be God, which hath not turned away my prayer,
nor his mercy from me.
Psalm 66:19 & 20

NOTES

_____

_____

_____

_____

_____

_____

_____

DAY 8

21 Day Weight Loss Challenge
SAMPLE Status Report

8AM   -   bottle of water

10AM   -   bottle of water

12PM   -   salad

2PM   -   bottle of water

4PM   -   soup

6PM   -   fruit smoothie

8PM   -   snack

_____

_____

_____

_____

_____

_____

_____

DAY 8

21 Day Weight Loss Challenge   -   Status Report

_____

_____

_____

_____

_____

_____

_____

_____

_____

_____

_____

_____

_____

_____

_____

DAY 9

21 Day Weight Loss Challenge
SAMPLE Status Report

8AM   -   bottle of water

10AM   -   bottle of water

12PM   -   salad

2PM   -   bottle of water

4PM   -   soup

6PM   -   green smoothie

8PM   -   snack

_____

_____

_____

_____

_____

_____

DAY 9

21 Day Weight Loss Challenge   -   Status Report

_____

_____

_____

_____

_____

_____

_____

_____

_____

_____

_____

_____

_____

DAY 10

21 Day Weight Loss Challenge
SAMPLE Status Report

8AM   -   bottle of water

10AM   -   bottle of water

12PM   -   salad

2PM   -   bottle of water

4PM   -   soup

6PM   -   fruit smoothie

8PM   -   snack

_____

_____

_____

_____

_____

_____

_____

DAY 10

21 Day Weight Loss Challenge   -   Status Report

_____

_____

_____

_____

_____

_____

_____

_____

_____

_____

_____

_____

_____

_____

_____

_____

DAY 11

21 Day Weight Loss Challenge
SAMPLE Status Report

8AM   -   bottle of water

10AM   -   bottle of water

12PM   -   salad

2PM   -   bottle of water

4PM   -   soup

6PM   -   lemonade

8PM   -   snack

_____

_____

_____

_____

_____

_____

_____

DAY 11

21 Day Weight Loss Challenge   -   Status Report

_____

_____

_____

_____

_____

_____

_____

_____

_____

_____

_____

_____

_____

_____

_____

DAY 12

21 Day Weight Loss Challenge
SAMPLE Status Report

8AM   -   bottle of water

10AM   -   bottle of water

12PM   -   salad

2PM   -   bottle of water

4PM   -   soup

6PM   -   lemonade

8PM   -   snack

_____

_____

_____

_____

_____

_____

_____

DAY 12

21 Day Weight Loss Challenge   -   Status Report

_____

_____

_____

_____

_____

_____

_____

_____

_____

_____

_____

_____

_____

_____

_____

DAY 13

21 Day Weight Loss Challenge
SAMPLE Status Report

8AM   -   bottle of water

10AM   -   bottle of water

12PM   -   small meal

2PM   -   bottle of water

4PM   -   salad

6PM   -   green smoothie

8PM   -   snack

_____

_____

_____

_____

_____

_____

DAY 13

21 Day Weight Loss Challenge   -   Status Report

_____

_____

_____

_____

_____

_____

_____

_____

_____

_____

_____

_____

_____

_____

_____

_____

DAY 14

21 Day Weight Loss Challenge
SAMPLE Status Report

8AM   -   bottle of water

10AM   -   bottle of water

12PM   -   small meal

2PM   -   bottle of water

4PM   -   salad

6PM   -   green smoothie

8PM   -   snack

_____

_____

_____

_____

_____

_____

_____

DAY 14

21 Day Weight Loss Challenge   -   Status Report

_____

_____

_____

_____

_____

_____

_____

_____

_____

_____

_____

_____

_____

_____

_____

WEEK 3

Stay encouraged! This is the last week of the the 21 Day Challenge. You have rededicated your life to God, and made a new commitment to pray more. Now it is time to press forward. Repeat this everyday...

I press toward the mark for the prize
of the high calling of God in Christ Jesus.
Philippians 3:14

Read 1 Samuel 30. David had to encourage himself. Sometimes, we may not have others around to give us encouragement. Call someone, everyday this week, to encourage them, and you will feel encouraged too!

NOTES

_____

_____

_____

_____

_____

_____

_____

DAY 15

21 Day Weight Loss Challenge
SAMPLE Status Report

8AM   -   bottle of water

10AM   -   bottle of water

12PM   -   salad

2PM   -   bottle of water

4PM   -   soup

6PM   -   fruit smoothie

8PM   -   snack

_____

_____

_____

_____

_____

_____

_____

DAY 15

21 Day Weight Loss Challenge   -   Status Report

_____

_____

_____

_____

_____

_____

_____

_____

_____

_____

_____

_____

_____

_____

_____

_____

_____

DAY 16

21 Day Weight Loss Challenge
SAMPLE Status Report

8AM   -   bottle of water

10AM   -   bottle of water

12PM   -   salad

2PM   -   bottle of water

4PM   -   soup

6PM   -   green smoothie

8PM   -   snack

_____
_____
_____
_____
_____
_____
_____

DAY 16

21 Day Weight Loss Challenge   -   Status Report

_____

_____

_____

_____

_____

_____

_____

_____

_____

_____

_____

_____

_____

_____

_____

DAY 17

21 Day Weight Loss Challenge
SAMPLE Status Report

8AM   -   bottle of water

10AM   -   bottle of water

12PM   -   salad

2PM   -   bottle of water

4PM   -   soup

6PM   -   fruit smoothie

8PM   -   snack

_____

_____

_____

_____

_____

_____

_____

DAY 17

21 Day Weight Loss Challenge   -   Status Report

_____

_____

_____

_____

_____

_____

_____

_____

_____

_____

_____

_____

_____

_____

_____

DAY 18

21 Day Weight Loss Challenge
SAMPLE Status Report

8AM   -   bottle of water

10AM   -   bottle of water

12PM   -   salad

2PM   -   bottle of water

4PM   -   soup

6PM   -   lemonade

8PM   -   snack

_____

_____

_____

_____

_____

_____

_____

DAY 18

21 Day Weight Loss Challenge   -   Status Report

_____
_____
_____
_____
_____
_____
_____
_____
_____
_____
_____
_____
_____
_____
_____
_____

DAY 19

21 Day Weight Loss Challenge
SAMPLE Status Report

8AM   -   bottle of water

10AM   -   bottle of water

12PM   -   salad

2PM   -   bottle of water

4PM   -   soup

6PM   -   lemonade

8PM   -   snack

_____

_____

_____

_____

_____

_____

_____

DAY 19

21 Day Weight Loss Challenge   -   Status Report

_____

_____

_____

_____

_____

_____

_____

_____

_____

_____

_____

_____

_____

_____

_____

_____

DAY 20

21 Day Weight Loss Challenge
SAMPLE Status Report

8AM   -   bottle of water

10AM   -   bottle of water

12PM   -   small meal

2PM   -   bottle of water

4PM   -   salad

6PM   -   green smoothie

8PM   -   snack

_____
_____
_____
_____
_____
_____
_____

DAY 20

21 Day Weight Loss Challenge   -   Status Report

_____

_____

_____

_____

_____

_____

_____

_____

_____

_____

_____

_____

_____

_____

_____

_____

DAY 21

21 Day Weight Loss Challenge
SAMPLE Status Report

8AM   -   bottle of water

10AM   -   bottle of water

12PM   -   small meal

2PM   -   bottle of water

4PM   -   salad

6PM   -   green smoothie

8PM   -   snack

_____

_____

_____

_____

_____

_____

DAY 21

21 Day Weight Loss Challenge   -   Status Report

_____

_____

_____

_____

_____

_____

_____

_____

_____

_____

_____

_____

_____

_____

_____

_____

RESOURCES

The Holy Bible

First Place
Celebrating Victory

In Touch
Daily Reading for Devoted Living

http://www.myhdiet.com/

createanewuhealthministry.com

createanewu@consultant.com

teachingbythespiritministries.org

MY TESTIMONY

I am so thankful and great-full to be alive and well, in 2015. However, I will never forget 2014. It was my wake up call. But let's back up about 20 years. I stopped eating pork about that time and several years after that, I also started to cut down on the amount of beef, chicken and turkey, that I was consuming. And I still was trying to lose weight but had no concern for my health or getting healthy.

In January 2014, I finally made a decision to really start losing weight. I went from 262 to 245 by May. Unfortunately, on Saturday, May24th, I started having really bad pains in my back, due to a fall I had earlier in that week.

By Sunday, my Pastor had to call an ambulance to take me to the emergency room. However, they sent me home with some pain pills and told me to lose some weight and get some exercise. When I woke up on Monday morning, I could not walk and the pain was getting worse.

By Thursday, I started losing control of my bladder and bowels, so my Pastor had to call for another ambulance to take me back to the same emergency room. And once again, the sent me home with more pain pills and told me again, to lose weight and get some exercise. I was not able to walk since Monday, so it was extremely hard for me to get in the car to return home. After my Pastor took me back home, it took over an hour for me to get out of the car and crawl from the car to the front door of the house.

The pain continued to get worse, and by Saturday, my Pastor had to call a third ambulance. When they arrived this time, my Pastor asked them to take me to Ben Taub County Hospital, but due to the new city ambulance laws, they were not allowed to take me that far.

Therefore, she had to get on the internet and find a private ambulance service that would take me across town, to Ben Taub. I arrived with an extremely high temperature and in extreme pain. They admitted me, late that night on May 31st, and I went home on June 14th, walking with a walker and now weighing 227. God used them to save my life.

After all that pain and suffering, I was still trying to lose more weight, but had no concern for my health or getting healthy. Little did I know that this was all a setup by God to get me healthy. Sometimes we have to feel "desperate" before we will see the light or take action.

In late November 2014, I saw the light. Only because, 2 months earlier, in September, I noticed that my health was no longer improving. Thanks to physical therapy twice a week, I went from the walker, to a cane, and was now walking on my own.

But, I still could not bend. If I dropped anything on the floor I could not pick it up, I had horrible cramps in my legs and hands, using the toilet was still a challenge and my short-term memory was badly impaired. And this was not all.

As stated above, in late November, I saw the light. Someone told me about a DVD course explaining how the body works when it has real food...which is healthy nutritious food. After watching those DVD's, I felt so convicted. I knew I owed it to my God, to be healthy. And I had now learned how eating healthy nutritious food helps the body God created, be healthy.

This was exciting news to me, because of all the ailments I now had, were due to the fall in May 2014. This is why I was so "desperate". I knew that it was now time for me to stop trying to lose weight and start trying to get healthy. And I was ready to do whatever I had to do, to make that happen.

I started on the Hallelujah Diet, in the middle of December 2014. Now, I feel like a new person. This gave me a hunger to not only learn even more about eating healthy, but also to share this knowledge with God's people. I felt lead to enrolled in the Certified Health Minister course, offered by Hallelujah Diet, and I graduated on March 20th.

I have learn how to make "tasty" but healthy meals. Learning to eat healthy is a life changing experience. It is not a fad or a diet. It is something that must be done for the rest of your life. I love waking up in the morning full of energy instead of tired and worn out before I even get out of bed. It feels so good to feel good!

This is a case of (the third time is the charm), because this journey took me up 3 levels. The first level of this journey was all about "ME" losing weight. And the second level was all about "ME" getting healthy. But now I know, that this journey has never been about me at all. It is and has always been, about GOD and rebuilding HIS temple, which is the third level.

WOW!!! What an eyeopener! I thank God! Now, instead of giving my "flesh" what it wants, I give my "body" what it needs, to rebuild the temple of God. Amen!

Dr. Kathleen B. Oden

Dr. Kathleen B. Oden

Dr. Kathleen B. Oden, is an author and Bible teacher that has been writing books and creating Bible games since 1998. She created Bible games, to help the children at her Church learn more about the Bible and have fun doing it. In 2012 she created a Hebrew Training Manual & Workbook, after taking a course in Hebrew, from the Hebrew University of Jerusalem. She has already used the manual, to teach private Hebrew lessons and it was her first published work.

Dr. Oden is currently working on a book called The Old Testament Synopsis, which will be published in 2016.

****

EDUCATION

1995-2000 - DEGREES:
Associate, Bachelor, Masters & Doctorate Degree
@ Immanuel Temple School of the Bible

2012 - HEBREW STUDIES:
HEBREW UNIVERSITY OF JERUSALEM
HOLY LANGUAGE INSTITUTE

2013 - TORAH STUDY:
TORAH CLASS - TOM BRADFORD

2015 - COMPLETED CERTIFICATION FOR HEALTH MINISTER:
HALLELUJAH ACRES TRAIN COURSE

2015 - FORMED: CREATE ANEWU HEALTH MINISTRY

****

LITERARY WORKS

1998   THE HOLY SPIRIT *(Masters Degree Thesis)*
2000   About The Bible *(Doctorate Degree Thesis)*
2004   The Old Testament *(Synopsis)*
2005   What God Commanded - *published:2015*
2006   The New Testament *(Synopsis)*
2010   Braggin About My God *(Poem)* - *published:2015*

2012 Who Is My Soulmate (Poem) - published:2015
2012 Hebrew Training Manual & Workbook - published:2015
2012 Hebrew Aleph-Bet Story & Workbook - published:2015
2012 Biblical Hebrew & Aleph-Bet Workbook - published:2015
2015 All About The Bible - published:2015
2015 21 Day Weight Loss Challenge & Workbook/Journal- published:2015
2015 Create Anewu Health Ministry Journal- published:2015
2015 Teaching By The Spirit Ministries Journal- published:2015

****

WEBSITES

http://www.teachingbythespiritministries.org/home.html

http://www.createanewuhealthministry.com/